Introduction

Losing weight can be a challenging and frustrating process, but with the right plan and mindset, it is possible to see results in just 30 days. In this book, we will outline a comprehensive plan for achieving your weight loss goals through diet and walking. We believe that this approach is not only effective but also safe and sustainable for long-term success.

The benefits of a 30-day plan: Research has shown that shorter-term goals can be more effective in achieving weight loss success than longer-term goals. By focusing on a 30-day timeframe, you can stay motivated and committed to your goals while also allowing yourself the flexibility to make adjustments to your plan as you go.

Additionally

The drawbacks of other approaches: Long-term diets and workout plans can be difficult to stick to, and the results may not be visible for months or even years. This can lead to frustration and feelings of failure, which can ultimately cause people to give up on their weight loss goals altogether.

Chapter 1:
Why 30 Days?

Losing weight can be a challenging and frustrating process, but it is essential for our overall health and well-being. Many people struggle with weight loss because they expect immediate results or do not have a clear plan to follow. That's why in this book, we will provide you with a 30-day plan to help you lose weight quickly and effectively.

But why 30 days? It's a reasonable time frame to

achieve noticeable results and establish healthy habits without overwhelming or exhausting yourself. You may be wondering why not 60 or 90 days, which might seem like a more significant amount of time. However, the 30-day period is long enough to see a visible difference and short enough to stay motivated and focused on your goals.

During these 30 days, you will learn how to make healthier choices, develop a better understanding of your body's needs, and establish sustainable habits that will help you maintain your weight loss progress in the long run. Additionally, setting a specific timeline will help you stay accountable, and you'll be more likely to stick to your plan if you have a clear goal in mind.

Another benefit of committing to a 30-day plan is that it can help you break the cycle of unhealthy habits that may have been holding you back from losing weight. Research shows that it takes about 21 days to form a new habit, so a 30-day plan gives you a bit of extra time to solidify these new habits.

It's essential to keep in mind that weight loss is a journey, and it takes time and effort to achieve your goals. By committing to a 30-day plan, you can jumpstart your weight loss journey and establish the foundation for a healthier lifestyle. With patience, determination, and consistency, you can achieve your desired results and maintain your progress in the long run.

Chapter 2: Understanding different weight loss approaches

Losing weight is a challenging task that requires commitment and hard work. However, with so many weight loss approaches available, it can be overwhelming to choose the right one. In this chapter, we will explore some of the most popular weight loss approaches and their advantages and disadvantages.

1. Low-calorie diets: Low-calorie diets involve reducing

your daily calorie intake to create a calorie deficit, which can lead to weight loss. These diets typically restrict or eliminate certain foods and focus on whole, nutrient-dense foods. The advantage of low-calorie diets is that they can lead to significant weight loss in a short amount of time. However, they can be difficult to sustain long-term, and some people may experience side effects such as hunger, fatigue, and nutrient deficiencies.

2. Low-carbohydrate diets: Low-carbohydrate diets involve reducing your carbohydrate intake and increasing your fat and protein intake. These diets aim to force your body into a state of ketosis, where it burns fat for energy instead of carbohydrates. The advantage of low-carbohydrate diets is that they can lead to rapid weight loss and improved blood sugar control. However, they can be difficult to sustain

long-term, and some people may experience side effects such as constipation, bad breath, and fatigue.

3. Intermittent fasting: Intermittent fasting involves alternating periods of eating and fasting. The most popular form of intermittent fasting is the 16/8 method, where you eat during an eight-hour window and fast for 16 hours. The advantage of intermittent fasting is that it can lead to weight loss, improved insulin

sensitivity, and reduced inflammation. However, it may not be suitable for everyone, and some people may experience side effects such as hunger, headaches, and dizziness.

4. Exercise: Exercise is an important component of any weight loss approach. It can help you burn calories, increase muscle mass, and improve overall health. The advantage of exercise is that it can lead to sustainable into

a busy schedule, and some people may experience injuries or discomfort.

5. Behavioral changes: Behavioral changes involve making small changes to your daily habits and routines to promote weight loss. Examples include tracking your food intake, practicing mindful eating, and getting enough sleep.The advantage of behavioral changes is that they can lead to sustainable weight loss and improved

overall health. However, they may not lead to rapid weight loss and may require significant effort and commitment.
After understanding the advantages and disadvantages of each weight loss approach, we will explain why our 30-day plan involves a combination of low-calorie diets and regular physical activity. . We believe that this approach is the most effective and sustainable for achieving rapid weight loss and

improving overall health. In the next chapter, we will provide a detailed plan for following this approach for 30 days.

Chapter 3: Weekly Action Plan

Now that you understand the benefits of a 30-day weight loss plan and have gained insight into different weight loss approaches, it's time to develop a weekly action plan to help you achieve your weight loss goals.

Week 1: During the first week, you'll focus on making small changes to your diet and physical activity levels. Start by eliminating unhealthy snacks and replacing them with healthier options, such as fruits, vegetables, or nuts.

Cut down on sugar and processed foods, and choose lean protein sources like chicken, fish, and legumes. To increase your physical activity, start with short walks or light cardio exercises for at least 20 minutes a day.

Week 2: In the second week, you'll ramp up your physical activity and continue making healthy food choices. Add strength training exercises to your routine to build muscle and increase your metabolism. Consider joining a fitness class or hiring a personal trainer for guidance. Also, focus on increasing your water intake and reducing your alcohol and caffeine consumption.

Week 3: During the third week, continue to increase your physical activity and focus on reducing your calorie intake. Start tracking your daily calorie intake and aim to create a calorie deficit of 500-1000 calories per day.

Eat more fiber-rich foods like fruits, vegetables, and whole grains to keep you feeling full for longer. Also, try to incorporate more high-intensity interval training (HIIT) into your workouts to maximize calorie burning.

Week 4: In the final week, maintain your healthy eating habits and continue to challenge yourself with intense workouts. Consider adding resistance training to your workouts to build muscle and increase your metabolism further. Evaluate your progress and celebrate your successes, no matter how small they may seem. Throughout the 30-day plan, it's essential to stay consistent and disciplined. Keep track of your progress, monitor your calorie intake and physical activity, and make adjustments as needed. Remember that everyone's body is different, so be patient with yourself and stay focused on your goals. By the end of the 30 days, you'll be amazed at how far you've come.

Chapter 4: Success Stories and Recommendations

One of the best ways to convince readers of the effectiveness of the 30-day weight loss plan is to include success stories and recommendations from individuals who have followed the plan and achieved significant results. In this chapter, we will share some of these stories and recommendations to inspire and motivate readers to stick to the plan and reach their weight loss goals.

Success Story 1: John's

Journey

John had struggled with his weight for years, trying different diets and exercise programs with little success. However, after following the 30-day weight loss plan, he was able to lose 15 pounds and drop two pants sizes. John was thrilled with his results and shared that he never felt hungry or deprived during the 30-day period

Success

Maria
Success
Sarah had tried many different diets and exercise programs in the past but always found herself gaining back the weight she had lost. However, after following the 30-day weight loss plan, Sarah not only lost 10 pounds but also learned sustainable habits that allowed her to maintain her weight loss long-term. She shared that the plan taught her to make healthier food choices and to

prioritize regular exercise, even after the 30-day period had ended.

Recommendations:

In addition to success stories, it is also helpful to include recommendations from professionals in the field of nutrition and weight loss. Here are some of the top recommendations for weight loss success:

1.Prioritize whole foods: Focus on consuming whole, nutrient-dense foods like fruits, vegetables, lean proteins, and healthy fats to promote satiety and overall health.

2.Stay hydrated: Drinking plenty of water can help reduce feelings of hunger and promote healthy digestion.

3.Incorporate strength training: Strength training can help build muscle mass, which can increase metabolism and promote fat loss.

4.Stay accountable: Whether it's through a supportive friend or a tracking app, find a way to hold yourself accountable to your weight loss goals.

By including success stories and recommendations, readers can see that the 30-day weight loss plan has worked for real people and has been endorsed by professionals in the field. This can help build trust in the plan and increase motivation to stick to it for the full 30 days.

Chapter 5: Bonuses and Add-Ons

Congratulations on making it this far in the 30-day weight loss plan! To help you achieve even greater success, we have put together a list of bonuses and add-ons that you can use to complement the diet and exercise plan.

1.Meal Delivery Services
Preparing healthy meals can be time-consuming and challenging for those with busy schedules. If you find it difficult to follow the diet plan because of lack of time,

consider using a meal delivery service. These services offer pre-made meals designed specifically for weight loss, taking the guesswork and effort out of meal planning and preparation. Additionally, most meal delivery services offer a variety of meal options to choose from, so you can pick the ones that align with your dietary restrictions and taste preferences.

2.Dietary Supplements

Dietary supplements can help support your weight loss journey by providing your body with essential nutrients that may be lacking in your diet. Some supplements, such as protein powders, can help keep you full and satiated, while others, such as multivitamins, can help ensure that you're getting all the necessary nutrients to support healthy weight loss. It's important to note that supplements should not be used as a substitute for a healthy diet, but rather as a complement to it.

3.Fitness Apps
If you find it challenging to motivate yourself to exercise, consider using a fitness app. These apps offer a variety of workouts and exercise routines that you can do at home or at the gym. They also provide you with the ability to track your progress and set achievable goals, which can help you stay

motivated and on track.

4.Personal Trainer
If you're not sure where to start with your exercise routine or want personalized guidance, consider hiring a personal trainer. A personal trainer can design a workout plan that aligns with your goals and fitness level, as well as provide you with guidance and motivation throughout your weight loss journey.

5.Support Groups
Joining a support group can be a helpful way to stay motivated and on track with your weight loss goals. Support groups offer a community of people who are going through similar experiences and can provide encouragement, advice, and accountability. Many support groups are available online, so you can participate from the comfort of your own home.

By using these bonuses and add-ons in conjunction with the diet and exercise plan, you can accelerate your weight loss journey and achieve even greater success. Remember, it's important to consult with your doctor before starting any new supplements or exercise routines.

Chapter 6: Maintaining Motivation

Losing weight is not an easy task, and it requires a lot of dedication and motivation. It's easy to start strong, but sticking with the program for 30 days can be challenging. In this chapter, we'll discuss some strategies to help you maintain your motivation throughout the 30-day program and beyond.

1.Regular progress checks: One of the best ways to stay motivated is to track your progress regularly. Set up a schedule to weigh yourself once a week, and take measurements of your waist, hips, and thighs. Seeing progress over time can be incredibly motivating and give you the momentum to continue with your program.

2.Celebrate milestones: Celebrating small milestones can be a great way to stay motivated. For example, if you hit your weight loss goal for the week, treat yourself to a non-food reward like a massage, a new outfit, or a movie. Celebrating small successes can help you feel good about your progress and keep you motivated to keep going.

3.Find a workout buddy: Having a workout buddy can help keep you accountable and make exercising more fun. You can motivate each other to keep going, and it can be helpful to have someone to talk to about the challenges you're facing.

4.Focus on non-scale victories: While weight loss is the primary goal, there are other benefits to eating healthy and exercising regularly. For example, you may notice that your energy levels have increased, your skin is clearer, or your clothes fit better. Celebrate these non-scale victories as well, as they can be incredibly motivating.

5.Stay positive: It's important to stay positive and avoid

negative self-talk. Remind yourself of the reasons why you started this program and focus on the progress you're making, rather than any setbacks or challenges you're facing.

6.Visualize success: Visualization can be a powerful tool for motivation. Take some time each day to visualize yourself at your goal weight and imagine how you'll feel when you get there. This can help you stay motivated and focused on your goal.

7.Stay flexible: Finally, it's important to stay flexible and be kind to yourself. There will be days when you don't meet your goals, and that's okay. Don't beat yourself up over it, just get back on track the next day. Remember that this is a marathon, not a sprint, and that slow progress is still progress.

By using these strategies, you can maintain your

motivation and stay on track with your weight loss goals throughout the 30-day program and beyond.

Chapter 7: Diet and Exercise Details

In this chapter, we'll take a closer look at the diet and exercise plan for the 30-day weight loss program. We'll provide you with specific details on the recommended diet, including meal plans and recipes, as well as a step-by-step exercise plan in the form of daily walks.

Diet Details:

To achieve the best results in weight loss, it is essential to maintain a balanced and healthy diet throughout the 30-day program.

We recommend a calorie-restricted diet that includes nutrient-rich foods such as lean proteins, fruits, vegetables, whole grains, and healthy fats.

We have designed a 30-day meal plan to help you stay on track with your diet. Here's a sample menu for the first week:

Day 1:

·Breakfast: Greek yogurt with mixed berries and almonds

·Snack: Apple slices with

almond butter
·Lunch: Grilled chicken salad with mixed greens, cherry tomatoes, cucumbers, and balsamic vinaigrette
·Snack: Carrots and hummus
·Dinner: Grilled salmon with quinoa and roasted asparagus

Day 2:
·Breakfast: Oatmeal with sliced banana and walnuts
·Snack: String cheese and grapes
·Lunch: Turkey and avocado

wrap with lettuce, tomato, and honey mustard dressing
·Snack: Pear slices with almond butter
·Dinner: Grilled shrimp with brown rice and roasted broccoli

Day 3:
·Breakfast: Veggie omelet with spinach, mushrooms, and onions
·Snack: Cherry tomatoes and mozzarella balls
·Lunch: Lentil soup with whole-grain bread

·Snack: Celery sticks and peanut butter
·Dinner: Baked chicken with sweet potato and green beans

Day 4:
·Breakfast: Greek yogurt with granola and sliced peaches
·Snack: Baby carrots and ranch dressing
·Lunch: Tuna salad with mixed greens, tomatoes, and cucumber
·Snack: Strawberries and whipped cream

·Dinner: Beef stir-fry with brown rice and mixed vegetables

Day 5:
·Breakfast: Banana and peanut butter smoothie
·Snack: Hard-boiled egg and celery sticks
·Lunch: Grilled chicken with quinoa and roasted vegetables
·Snack: Blueberries and almonds
·Dinner: Baked salmon with mixed vegetables and

brown rice

Day 6:
·Breakfast: Scrambled eggs with spinach and feta cheese
·Snack: Cottage cheese with pineapple chunks
·Lunch: Grilled chicken Caesar salad with whole-grain croutons
·Snack: Apple slices with cinnamon
·Dinner: Turkey meatballs with spaghetti squash and marinara sauce

Day 7:
·Breakfast: Whole-grain toast with avocado and tomato
·Snack: Edamame
·Lunch: Greek salad with grilled chicken, feta cheese, and olives
·Snack: Mango slices
·Dinner: Grilled steak with roasted potatoes and green beans

Exercise Plan:
Physical activity is an essential component of the 30-day weight loss program.

We recommend at least 30 minutes of moderate-intensity exercise each day, in the form of brisk walking. Here is a step-by-step exercise plan for 30 days:

Week 1:

·Day 1-3: Walk for 15 minutes at a moderate pace

·Day 4: Rest

·Day 5-7: Walk for 20 minutes at a moderate pace

Week 2:

·Day 8-10: Walk for 25 minutes at a moderate pace

·Day 11: Rest

·Day 12-14: Walk for 30 minutes at a moderate pace

Week 3:

·Day 15-17: Walk for 35 minutes at a moderate pace

·Day 18: Rest

·Day 19-21: Walk for 40 minutes at a moderate pace

Week 4:

·Day 22-24: Walk for 45 minutes at a moderate pace

·Day 25: Rest

·Day 26-28: Walk for 50 minutes at a moderate pace

·Day 12-14: Walk for 30 minutes at a moderate pace

Week 3:

·Day 15-17: Walk for 35 minutes at a moderate pace

·Day 18: Rest

·Day 19-21: Walk for 40 minutes at a moderate pace

Week 4:

·Day 22-24: Walk for 45 minutes at a moderate pace

·Day 25: Rest

·Day 26-28: Walk for 50 minutes at a moderate pace

Week 5:

·Day 29-30: Walk for 60

minutes at a moderate pace It's important to remember to warm up before and cool down after each walk. Start with a slow pace and gradually increase your speed as you feel comfortable. You can also add in some strength training exercises, such as lunges or squats, to your routine to help build muscle and boost your metabolism.

Overall, the combination of a healthy, balanced diet and

regular exercise will help you achieve your weight loss goals and maintain a healthy lifestyle. Remember to stay motivated and dedicated to the program, and don't hesitate to reach out for support or guidance if needed.

Chapter 8: How Diet and Exercise Affect Weight Loss

In this chapter, we'll take a deeper look at the relationship between diet, exercise, and weight loss. Understanding how these factors work together can help you make the most out of your 30-day weight loss program.

Diet and Weight Loss:

Diet is a crucial factor in weight loss. To lose weight, you must create a calorie deficit, which means consuming fewer calories than your body burns.

This can be achieved through a combination of reducing calorie intake and increasing physical activity.

When it comes to weight loss, not all calories are created equal. For example, a calorie from a donut is not the same as a calorie from a chicken breast. The quality of the calorie matters, as well as the quantity. It is essential to focus on nutrient-dense foods that provide your body with the vitamins and minerals it needs to function optimally.

Processed and high-sugar foods should be limited as they provide empty calories that do not provide much nutritional value. Instead, choose foods such as lean proteins, fruits, vegetables, whole grains, and healthy fats, as these provide your body with the nutrients it needs while helping you feel full and satisfied.

Exercise and Weight Loss: Exercise is another essential factor in weight loss. It helps to burn calories and build lean muscle mass, which increases your metabolism and helps you burn more calories even when you're not exercising.

Aerobic exercise, such as walking, jogging, or cycling, is an effective way to burn calories and lose weight. Resistance training, such as lifting weights, can also be beneficial in building muscle mass and increasing metabolism.

It's important to note that exercise alone is not enough to achieve significant weight loss. A combination of diet and exercise is necessary to create a calorie deficit and lose weight effectively.

The Bottom Line:

In conclusion, both diet and exercise are essential components of weight loss. To achieve the best results, it's essential to maintain a calorie-restricted diet that includes nutrient-rich foods while engaging in regular physical activity. Remember that weight loss is a journey, and small changes over time can lead to significant improvements in your health and well-being.

Chapter 9: Exercise Examples and Instructions

In this chapter, we'll provide you with examples of exercises that you can incorporate into your daily routine to enhance your weight loss journey. It's essential to keep in mind that physical activity is not only beneficial for weight loss, but it also improves your overall health and well-being.

Here are some exercises you can try:

1.Squats: Squats are an excellent exercise for building leg muscles and improving balance. Stand with your feet shoulder-width apart, and then lower your hips back and down as if you are sitting in a chair. Keep your weight in your heels and your chest lifted. Lower down until your thighs are parallel to the ground, then return to standing.

2.Push-ups: Push-ups are a classic exercise for building upper body strength. Start in a plank position with your hands slightly wider than shoulder-width apart. Lower your body down, bending your elbows until your chest almost touches the ground, then push back up to the starting position.

3.   Lunges: Lunges are another great exercise for building leg muscles and improving balance. Start with your feet hip-width apart, and then step forward with one foot. Bend both knees, lowering your body until your front thigh is parallel to the

ground, and your back knee is hovering above the floor. Push through your front heel and step back to the starting position. Repeat on the other side.

4.Jumping Jacks: Jumping jacks are an excellent cardiovascular exercise that gets your heart pumping. Start with your feet together and your arms at your sides. Jump your feet out and raise your arms overhead, then jump back to the starting position.

5.Planks: Planks are a great exercise for strengthening your core muscles. Start in a push-up position, then lower down onto your forearms. Keep your body in a straight line from your head to your heels, and hold for as long as you can.

Instructions:
It's essential to perform each

exercise correctly to prevent injury and maximize its effectiveness. Here are some tips for performing each exercise:

1.Squats: Keep your weight in your heels, your chest lifted, and your knees tracking over your toes.

2.Push-ups: Keep your body in a straight line from your head to your heels, and lower your body down until your chest almost touches the ground.

3.Lunges: Keep your front knee tracking over your toes, your weight in your front heel, and your chest lifted.

4.Jumping Jacks: Keep your arms and legs straight, and jump with control.

5.Planks: Keep your body in a straight line from your head to your heels, and engage your core muscles by pulling your belly button toward your spine.

Conclusion:
Incorporating these exercises

into your daily routine can help you achieve your weight loss goals and improve your overall health and well-being. Remember to perform each exercise correctly to prevent injury, and gradually increase the intensity and duration of your workouts as you progress. Consult with a doctor before starting any new exercise routine, especially if you have any pre-existing health conditions.

Chapter 10: Mental Health and Weight Loss

In this chapter, we will focus on the importance of mental health in weight loss. While diet and exercise are crucial in achieving weight loss goals, the role of mental health should not be underestimated. Weight loss can be a challenging journey, and one's mental health can play a significant role in their ability to succeed.

One of the most important aspects of mental health in weight loss is the ability to manage stress. When we experience stress, our bodies release the hormone cortisol, which can trigger cravings for high-fat, high-sugar foods. This can lead to overeating, making weight loss more challenging.

To manage stress, it's essential to practice stress-reducing techniques, such as mindfulness meditation, yoga, or deep breathing exercises. Engaging in regular physical activity can also be an effective way to reduce stress and boost mood.

Another critical aspect of mental health in weight loss is self-compassion. Many people tend to be hard on themselves when they experience setbacks or struggle to meet their weight loss goals. This can lead to feelings of guilt and shame, which can further hinder progress.

To promote self-compassion, it's important to treat oneself with kindness, understanding, and acceptance. This means avoiding self-criticism and focusing on the positive aspects of one's weight loss journey, no matter how small they may be.

Another way to promote mental health in weight loss is to stay motivated and engaged in the process. This can be achieved by setting realistic and achievable goals, tracking progress, and celebrating small victories along the way. It's also important to stay accountable by enlisting the support of friends, family members, or

a weight loss support group. Lastly, it's essential to remember that weight loss is not a one-size-fits-all process. Everyone's journey is unique, and it's important to approach weight loss with an open mind and a willingness to adapt as needed. This means finding a diet and exercise plan that works for one's individual needs and preferences, and being flexible enough to adjust as circumstances change.
In conclusion,

mental health is a crucial component of weight loss. By managing stress, practicing self-compassion, staying motivated and engaged, and being open to change, one can achieve their weight loss goals and maintain a healthy lifestyle.

Chapter 11: Healthy Snack Ideas

Snacking can be an essential part of any weight loss program, as it can help keep your hunger in check between meals and prevent overeating. However, not all snacks are created equal, and it's essential to choose healthy options that provide essential nutrients while keeping calories in check. In this chapter, we'll share some healthy snack ideas that are both satisfying and good for you.

1.Greek Yogurt with Berries: Greek yogurt is an excellent source of protein and calcium, and adding fresh berries can add sweetness and fiber to your snack. Choose plain, unsweetened yogurt to keep the calorie count low, and top with your favorite berries.

2.Hard-Boiled Eggs: Hard-boiled eggs are a great source of protein and healthy fats, and they're easy to prepare ahead of time and take on-the-go. Sprinkle some salt and pepper on top for added flavor.

3.Hummus and Vegetables: Hummus is a delicious dip made from chickpeas and tahini, and it pairs well with crunchy vegetables like carrots, cucumbers, and bell peppers. This snack is low in calories and high in fiber and protein, making it an excellent choice for weight loss.

4.Apple Slices with Almond Butter: Apples are high in fiber and antioxidants, and pairing them with almond butter provides healthy fats and protein. This snack is satisfying and delicious, perfect for curbing your sweet cravings.

5.Air-Popped Popcorn: Popcorn can be a healthy snack choice when prepared correctly. Air-popped popcorn is low in calories and high in fiber, making it a great option for weight loss. Avoid pre-packaged microwave popcorn, which can be high in calories and unhealthy fats.

6.Cottage Cheese with

Pineapple: Cottage cheese is high in protein and calcium, and pairing it with fresh pineapple provides natural sweetness and vitamin C. This snack is satisfying and low in calories, perfect for any time of day.

7.Edamame: Edamame is a type of soybean that is high in protein and fiber, and it makes for an excellent snack. Simply steam or boil edamame and sprinkle with some salt for a healthy and satisfying snack.

8.Roasted Chickpeas: Chickpeas are a great source of protein and fiber, and roasting them can add crunch and flavor. Toss cooked chickpeas with some olive oil and your favorite spices, and roast in the oven for a tasty and healthy snack.

9.Fruit Salad: A fruit salad is a delicious and refreshing snack that can provide a variety of essential vitamins and minerals. Combine your favorite fruits, such as berries, melons, and citrus, for a healthy and satisfying snack.

10.Turkey Roll-Ups: Turkey roll-ups are an easy and tasty snack that provides protein and healthy fats. Simply roll a slice of turkey around a piece of avocado or cucumber for a low-calorie snack that will keep you full and satisfied.

Incorporating these healthy snack ideas into your weight loss program can help keep your hunger in check and provide essential nutrients to .

support your weight loss
goals. Remember to keep
portion sizes in mind, and
choose snacks that are low in
calories and high in nutrients

Conclusion

In conclusion, the 30-day weight loss program can be a highly effective way to achieve your weight loss goals. By following the diet and exercise plan provided in this guide, you can create a sustainable lifestyle that promotes healthy habits and a positive mindset.

Remember, weight loss is not just about achieving a number on the scale. It is about improving your overall health and well-being, both physically and mentally. This program is designed to help you achieve both of these goals.

Throughout the 30-day program, it's important to track your progress and celebrate your successes, no matter how small they may seem. Remember that weight loss is a journey, and it's normal to experience setbacks and challenges along the way. The key is to stay motivated and committed

to your goals.
By incorporating healthy habits into your daily routine and maintaining a positive mindset, you can achieve long-term success in your weight loss journey. Good luck on your journey to a healthier you!